Smart Body

The Skin You Exist Within

Carrington Allen

This edition first published in 2022
Carrington Allen
www.carringtonallen.com

ISBN 978-1-387-78995-5

Printed in the United States of America

ACKNOWLEDGEMENTS

Thank you to Source for continued messages of clarity and guidance. I feel honored to be trusted with these words to share with you.

Thank you to my children and my mother for their support over the past few months. Matthew for your inspirational smile and kindness, thought provoking questions, and out-of-the-box perceptions. Emily for your guidance in editing, your readiness to always lend a hand to anyone in need, and your gentle fierceness that keeps you balanced when others stumble. Sophie for your vision to see the unseen, your creative reasoning, and your stubborn but strong sense of self. And my mom, thank you for your unending amount of time to just listen as I share so much information, for welcoming us into your home whenever we popped into town, and for the years of love and compassion you showered us all with. These books would not be possible without their support. These are the souls I call my family and am honored to have them close to my heart.

This book is written for those
that are just beginning the
journey of understanding
their physical presence and the
essence that resides within.

Dear Reader,

This book is written as one long letter from Source to you. You are the soul that is on the journey home surrounded by distractions that keep you from living your best life.

Just like my other books, this one was given to me from Source through the same process. I sit and type the thoughts that come streaming into my head. And then, I pause and ask if I have captured them correctly. I also see visions and gain other information that accompany these words. It is difficult to explain, but there are many levels to each sentence that is received. We have a very fast conversation of sorts that moves faster than I could ever expect to type or speak. The extra information is given to me to help me understand in greater detail what is being shared.

I do wish I had the ability to convey everything that is given, but I hope that these words will help you gain a greater understanding of the physical body and the power you have over your health and well-being as well as your life path.

Thank you,
Carrington

Your letter from Source...

Dear One,

Your soul, spirit, and ego mind are all within this shell, your smart body.

Now, what makes it smart? Is it your ego mind?

Your ego mind is in charge of the daily activities.

These include breathing, blood and oxygen circulation, and physical activities such as walking, reading, and listening. So, there is a purpose for the ego mind. It also helps protect what we will refer to the physical body as the SB (smart body).

You could say the SB is the outer shell of a computer or robot. And the ego mind is the software that runs it. This information is expanded by all of the bits of information you are exposed to through your observation of movies, books, other people, etc. During your entire life, you are gathering information to be used in this software system to "make decisions" based on what you have perceived.

A note at this point is that all decisions made with the guidance of the ego mind are derived from perceptions gathered from all of your past experiences. These decisions are not guided by divine reality or divine knowledge.

Another note to make is that your ego mind does not have the ability to guide you in terms of morality or benevolence. It does not understand the difference between what is right and what is wrong.

The ego mind does not love. It only grabs information and stores it and brings it to the surface to remind you of the past. It brings forth the good and the bad memories. And therefore, it is the producer of the emotion of guilt.

And here is the interesting thing. The ego mind is the producer of information to help you analyze situations. It creates a mental environment for you to compare and contrast information to help you decide what to do – but it is based entirely upon bits of information gathered, unrelated at the time to this decision and without the big picture being available to be seen. How can you make a decision with these blinders on? And with only partial information? But yet, you do. Over and over again you rely on the ego mind to help you decide. And often you make bad choices based on this information.

When you realize what has happened, you often feel guilty about your choice. Is this your fault? Do you deserve the guilt? What if you were to rely on another Source and accept the guidance from this Source that is always choosing for the highest good?

You would never make a bad or negative choice again. Period. Guilt would no longer exist in your life.

What happens when you feel badly about something that has transpired in your life? Well, I will tell you, you develop a pattern of emotions that present themselves to you over and over again. Yes, for the same event, you can create this pattern that will run over and over like a bad movie in your mind, and this is what generates the emotions. Once these emotions have been created, they can't be destroyed. They can only be transmuted because thoughts and emotions are energy. Just like you are an energetic being, these emotions can meld together to create spaces in your physical body, appearing to have taken on physical form. Often labeled as tumors or other blockages, these balls or spheres of energy can wreak havoc on your system by blocking the flow of energy needed to keep your body healthy.

Every cell within your body is connected not only physically but also in terms of communication. When your emotions send out an energetic vibe, that energy travels and is communicated to each and every cell. When the energy is flowing freely, it does not become trapped and eventually is flushed out of your system. But when there is not enough oxygen or water to help carry this energy through, it can become stuck, and once one energetic atom becomes lodged, others will attach, causing a type of coagulation that creates a blockage. These blockages impede the flow of energy, including everything your body needs to stay well (nutrients for cell repair, water for energy flow, etc.).

Learning how to avoid having these emotional energies coagulating is the beginning to your road back to health and wellness. Your physical body is the outer shell, the casing for your soul. Like a computer with software (the ego mind), it will occasionally need maintenance. Ridding the physical body of these negative energies frees up the space and pathways for your energy to regulate and maintain your bodily functions. And this keeps you in top physical form to house your soul and live a vibrant, healthy long life.

Sometimes cells break down on their own without the influence of emotional trappings. This can be caused by the exposure to harsh toxins and chemicals, dissonant sounds, and other unhealthy substances that are often ingested. When this is the cause of the cells disintegrating, you will need to focus your intentions clearly on communicating to your innate body to repair these structures and bring them back into balance. The power that you have through your thoughts and intentions is unlimited. You are a creator, and you create everything within your physical and non-physical world.

For example, if you constantly talk to friends and family and share what is "wrong with you," you are setting the stage for illness for yourself. The cells in your body can literally receive this communication and take direction from it. If you proclaim yourself to be sick, then that is what you will be. Very simple, yet often ignored, you are what you think you are.

Just like sticky cotton candy practically melts in your

mouth, energy changes form too. When sticky negative energy grasps on to other parts of your physical body, like sticky cotton candy, it becomes an unwanted residue. And as it builds like plaque on your teeth, it creates a harmful micro environment in your system. Since you are unable to reach deep within your physical body with a tool to remove the residue, you must discover another way to move that energy away from you, as you now understand how harmful it can be.

So, what should you do to remove it? It is as simple as setting the intention and energetically waving away these clumps of coagulated low vibrational energy. Since they are moving at such a slow vibrational pace, when you increase your overall vibration (raise your frequency), your overall energy will shake the stagnant energy loose, and it should be set free.

Moving from stagnant energy to the vibration of words and their effect on your body, whispering words communicate in a much more loving way than loud, booming voices. The effects of sound on your system are enormous. Think of a time that a loud noise practically pushed you out of your skin – perhaps it frightened you or just jarred you. You probably could actually feel the loud energy if it was absorbed in slow motion. Thank goodness it wasn't.
Every sound that you come in contact with tries to penetrate your protective outer energetic boundary. Many refer to this as your aura, an energy field that surrounds your body and attempts to filter out the negative "noise" and other detrimental toxic energy that flows your way.

I bet you had no idea that this outer layer of energy even existed for such a purpose. Many like to try and figure out the color of their aura, but they hardly understand its purpose.

The point of this information is to begin to outline your levels of protection. It starts with your aura that is closest to you and extends out to your Merkaba, which is more like a sphere of energy that extends out approximately 6 feet around you on all sides. The higher your energy is vibrating, the more it extends outward. And the lower your vibration, well, the smaller the sphere becomes, contracting and giving you less of a protective insulator space around you. As you can imagine, the more insulation you have, the better protected you are from all types of harmful energies.

An example of this might be if you are extremely happy to attend a concert, the noise will not seem as potent or jarring. But if you have been unwillingly coerced into attending a concert and are miserable, with a low vibration, you may leave with a headache or other physical symptoms. These symptoms are a result of the constant barrage of loud noises that gained easier access to your physical body due to a lack of greater insulation that would have been provided with a higher vibrational attitude.

With this knowledge beginning to grow about the importance of vibration, you will be able to begin to create a better atmosphere for your own well-being.

Levels are a way of measuring frequencies, and the different levels have different manifestation properties. Something of a low frequency is more dense and slow-moving, meaning it barely vibrates. In fact, to the physical sight, you can't even see it moving. As the frequency changes and the energy/atoms move more quickly, the energy becomes less dense. Your body is a combination of frequencies held together by light. I can hear your thoughts, *what? Light? How can that be?* What I am referring to is light energy, this is the frequency of love. The ultimate pure divine light is what holds everything together, and this is how we are all connected.

Can you visualize it? Try the image of a clear soup that fills every space that an atom does not fill. The space is so tiny that even under a microscope, your eyes can still not detect it. This is love. Love is everything and nothing.

So, what does this mean? Other than the fact that you are held together by My frequency, meaning you are held together by Source? Well, that sums it up.

But let's give your mind a break. We were focusing on the topic of your smart body in order that you might gain wisdom to heal whatever ailments you think that you have.

Hypnotic states of being are a time when your ego mind is totally in charge. Your physical body responds to direction while your soul removes itself from the chaos to be free to communicate with you on a higher level. It is as if the ego mind feels that it has been given full control, but it is only given control over how your physical body reacts to direction and therefore only has what you may consider half control. The soul, on the other hand, is free to quietly observe and download information to share with your mind. These may be represented as thought forms or may appear as visions, dreamlike pictures that you see. Sometimes these are animated partially or fully, and often they are just symbols to try and inspire a bit of information to be understood.

When you are physically still in a hypnotic state, your soul becomes not the observer but the influencer. It then gains full control and can relay information from your energetic being that is fully aware to your mind that is installed in your physical body. It can be a pathway to communicate with your soul.

Why is this important? This is where your true divine guidance is derived. It needs a pathway that is not interrupted by your ego mind. Your imagination is not a form of your ego mind, it is a link to the divine where wonderful ideas are shared with you, ideas to create new and exciting thoughts that may be turned into creations from the heart in physical form. The ego creates from information gathered and regurgitated. It is not new, nor is it creative. Stagnant ideas that are redundant and stale are from the ego mind. Now it sounds harsh to describe these in this manner, but it is important to see and understand the vast difference between what is derived from the ego mind and what is allowed to pass through to you from your divine connection.

And what passes through this divine connection other

than guidance? Often the ability to heal your mind, and therefore heal your physical body, is possible through this pathway if left free from obstruction.

Do you need to be in a hypnotic state for healing? Well, it helps. Some call it a meditative state, and that might more accurately describe it. But giving your soul the opportunity to call the shots will enable quicker healing of the physical body. By giving the soul a way to communicate clearly without obstruction with the mind that acts as a software-type program for the body, it enables the mind to clearly communicate what is needed to heal.

Walls are created in your mind to separate or protect yourself. Sometimes these are walls made of rules or boundaries that you or someone else create to make you think you are making your life easier. By boxing yourself in with rules, you often feel that you are simplifying your life by limiting your choices. The funny or ironic part of this behavior is that although in duality you have choices, there is only one best answer. No matter the situation, there is only one answer that fits the highest good for all. So, to live your best life and only live your truth should be simple.

But you can see the wrong answer or choice in duality. It sits there right in front of you, available to be chosen, a temptation. Somewhere in your heart, you know it is not the best choice. But you look around, and if others are choosing it, or you can somehow justify choosing it, you do.

And then many of you caught in the web of man-made religious practices call this sin. Is it though? It was just a choice, an error made. To correct the error, you just pivot and go in the opposite direction by choosing the better choice. And there is no reason for forgiveness, there is no sin, just error. Error easily corrected.

And what does this have to do with healing? It is the foundation for healing. First you must accept and create space for dismissal of errors. You must allow yourself to accept that you are good. You are love, and you are light. As long as you hold onto the thoughts that box you in as imperfect, you will never see yourself as whole and healed. By seeing yourself as anything less than how you were originally created is to give space to the illusion that you could actually be less than, or in your terms, ill.

And if you see yourself as less than whole, then how can you see Me, Source, as whole? You were created in My image, therefore you are whole. I can only see you as whole, and it is time for you to accept my image of you. Suffering is your own manifestation – a creation from your ego mind that only exists because it is substantiated by data collected during your lifetime. Your ego mind calls up this data to project to you to create an image of yourself that is only a projection, an illusion based on bits of information collected from the past. Standing in this moment accepting illusions of past traumas/events that no longer exist is what you have been basing your current moment on – and it is only an illusion. The true you that exists is whole and magnificent and eternal.

So, in this moment, allow yourself the privilege given as a gift from Me to let go of the illusions. Let go of the you created by your ego mind. To truly find yourself, you need only to let go of the illusion of yourself. The true you, the divinely inspired you is a creative soul waiting for the opportunity to live and create and extend all of your gifts out into the world. Sharing your gifts of peace and joy will be the beginning to not only healing yourself, but you will begin to heal the world. One smile at a time, dissolving the heartache that abounds, you will inspire others. And like dominos, your energy will extend out, touching people around the world. It starts with you. Healing yourself is the beginning to healing the world.

And is it easy? Not really, because you have become acquainted with not only a lifestyle here on Earth, but also with programming done by years of manipulation. These ways of controlling yourself and others have become your normal. This untangling from the web of ways learned and lived will be a challenging part of your journey. So many tools have been used to distract and manipulate your mind to work solo without consulting with your soul. And for some the disconnect is so strongly felt that it may seem they will never figure things out. You may have friends or family members that you want to help – you see them struggling, and you feel that you have the answers.

Please know, other than planting seeds, they are on their own journey. The best way to help another is to exemplify goodness, happiness, peace, and joy. And this doesn't mean to fake it. This means, for you to do the work, the hard work.

Now back to that physical body, the smart body.

What makes it so smart?

Your link, your channel, your connection to Me.

This connection gives you access to the ultimate guidance, the answer to every question, and the emotional support of a spiritual coach that is only invested in what is best for you and your family of souls that are connected to you through Me.

What more could you ask for?

Perhaps stability?
Peace in your life?
Everlasting joy?

Oh, but these are the gifts that are yours at the very moment that you extend them to others.

Think about this for just a moment. Peace is never yours when you are acting disruptive, rude, or deceitful. But when you extend peace from your heart sincerely, peace reverberates back to you.

Now, there are exceptions. But if you are consistent with extending the gift of peace and joy to others, you will most definitely find that you will be more often than not the recipient of peace and joy. And the more of you that are inspired to share this gift with others, the greater the results will be among you.

Now on to other topics – energy, frequency, and vibration. These are the keys to outlining the basics of your smart body. You understand that your body is composed of energy. Made of atoms that cluster together to create your physical body. But do you understand how the atoms are different? What makes them act or appear as certain aspects, for example, your lungs versus your brain? This is where you will need to begin to understand frequency.

Each atom within your body operates on a different frequency, and the frequency it operates within determines how it looks, feels, and acts. For example, the heart consisting of atoms resonates with a particular frequency of instructions. These instructions maintain its shape and function at all times unless the frequency is blocked by negative energy. What you consider negative energy, whether it is toxic chemicals or emotions of fear, vibrate at such a slow rate that they coagulate and clog channels of communication that are needed to receive the proper frequency information to provide wellness.

And this brings us to the importance of the vibrational rate of energy. As you can see when blockages occur, frequencies are blocked, and a breakdown of the organ or system begins. The easiest and most direct way to wellness is to break down those clogging energies and free the channels of communication. This is done by increasing the overall vibration of the physical body. Once the vibration is high, the blocked areas vibrate at a rate that can not be withstood by the lower, denser vibrating energy, and the blockage is shaken loose to be moved along out of the body.

So together, energy, frequency, and vibration determine your overall health and well-being. Consisting of nothing but energy in the form of atoms, you must set the intentions daily to cleanse your system of any blockages. Even if you are able to stay at a fairly high rate of vibration, your body will still absorb toxic energies that will form blockages. This is why healing methods including sound (to adjust frequencies), light (to adjust vibration), and color (to adjust overall energy) are most responsive to induce a return to health.

NOTE: Color projected onto yourself as it appears in your surroundings creates a reaction inducing emotions that can create a positive vibrational increase or a lower, denser response.

The exposure to sunlight enhances your ability to not only see more clearly but also to lower any fear response. Your body also absorbs many positive nutrients from the sun which makes positive adjustments to your cells' response to toxins and other emotional triggers.

The system is quite simple. Each part of you consists of a different frequency. In order to repair or re-create a part of you, you need only identify that frequency and apply it to the area in need of adjustment. Think of each part within you singing a song from a different radio station. If you cut off the music by changing the station, that one part will be lost and unable to continue singing the song as easily as before. When each part of you is able to clearly receive its frequency, it thrives just like you would be able to clearly hear the radio station without static or interruption.

Your ego mind helps regulate the frequencies by following the original blueprint that is ingrained within it. At any time, you can request your innate body to return to its original blueprint with all frequencies aligned and all blockages cleared. This will help your physical body stay maintained and well.

And now you ask, how do you estimate the appropriate frequencies that are needed for each part of yourself when you seek to repair something?

This is the interesting part. You only need to ask. Within your DNA, all of the appropriate instructions, guidelines, blueprints, etc. are stored, and your ego mind has access to this information. Your ego mind as the software of your body just needs your green light "go" request to enable the communication to begin. This is why I have referred to your body as the "smart body." It already knows what to do with such frequency requests, but until now you have not known that you needed to do this.

It is as simple as speaking aloud and stating: "Innate body, return all frequencies to the original blueprint formula to create a strong, well-balanced, aligned physical body." Simple. Just like that, over time your body will regenerate cells and will become well again.

But you should know there are ways that you tend to hinder the alignment and regenerated health. To start, your thoughts are much more powerful than you know, and your spoken words have the ability to wreak havoc on not only yourself but others.

For example, when you think or speak, "I am not well, I must be sick." You have just put in a call to every cell within your body alerting them that you are sick. And so, they now create the symptoms to match what you have stated because after all, you call the shots.

Or perhaps, when you say, "I always seem to have a sore throat." This causes an alert to be made that you have a sore throat. The same with... "I am tired." Or, "My eyes can't see very well." And, "I don't want to hear that!" creates problems with your hearing. BE CAREFUL WHAT YOU SAY. Because that is what you become.

Instead focus your thoughts on what is feeling great. My legs are so strong. I have so much energy today! I feel great! My lungs are powerful! I think you get the message.

Beyond thoughts, you may have the tendency to further sabotage your well-being by inhaling toxic chemicals from your environment or from "smoking" inhalants such as tobacco, or what you describe as other "medicinal" drugs.

And the list continues with the intake of toxic chemicals including alcohol, caffeine, and sugar.

Face it, in order to accomplish your goal of a well-balanced physical body, you will need to consider all areas of your life. And depending on your level of commitment, you will either have perfect health or not.

Perhaps you were looking for a quick fix. Maybe you think you need a personal coach to follow you around day after day to help you make the best choices. What if I told you this is provided for you from the first moment you acknowledge your inner guidance and begin to listen and follow it. You know the guidance, when you start to choose candy over a piece of fruit. Your inner guidance explicitly gives you the thoughts that the fruit is the better choice, but you don't follow it, and you choose the candy.

You have the inner guidance/coach always with you striving for your best outcome. Perhaps it's time that you gave it a chance. Try the 30-day challenge to follow that inner guidance for one month with every choice you make. If you did this, you would be shocked at how much your life would improve. This benevolent guidance waits for you to tune in and follow its path created for you to reach your best life.

What if? What if you took the challenge? I dare you.

When it's time to make decisions, to choose it is always simple. There is usually only one best choice. And you know deep within which one to choose. But often you choose the more tempting food, person, book, etc. Why is that?

What makes you think choosing something other than the best for you will make you happy? It might bring happiness for a few moments, but if you begin to think past the moment into the future, you will begin to see how the best choice is the only choice for happiness.

The bright and shiny choice that glitters now will become dull and boring when you realize it is without substance. And substance is what the soul thrives upon.

The illusions that come before you fade quickly once they pass through the energy of your physical body. They dissolve into nothing, whereas when you choose something of value, meaning, and authenticity, it lasts a lifetime and may create a favorable memory that will last eternally.

Choose substance over frivolity. Choose happiness over trying to impress someone else. Be authentic, be present, just be. A smart body has the ability to run itself, but the soul will need direction. For your soul's eternal stake in the everlasting, choose substance. Always choose substance.

At times you may feel that your head is filled with so many ideas at one time that you are unable to process any of them. This leads to not only confusion but exhaustion. The importance of clearing your thoughts is paramount in being able to allow your smart body to focus on exactly what it needs to in order to maintain your health and well-being.

Have you heard of meditation? Simply, this is the process of clearing your thoughts to allow for a better connection of sorts. And this will enhance your ability to focus on exactly what truly needs to be in your thoughts minus all the trivial things that truly do not matter.

Now to begin to practice this process may seem like a difficult task to those that have not experienced the pure pleasure of relaxing into the moment and just existing. Nothing more and nothing less – just being. With practice this process will become something that you will look forward to each day because you will experience the benefits and crave more. This is natural to crave more alone time to dismantle the web of information that you have become tangled within. It is not lazy to prioritize yourself first. If you do not spend the time to align and balance yourself, then you will be less than capable of fulfilling your own dreams or assisting anyone else. Taking time to breathe and clear your thoughts enables you to become present and fully whole in order to take on the day. Your smart body needs this time to reset.

Which brings us to the topic of sleep. While you sleep, your ego mind has the opportunity to focus entirely on running the systems of your physical body including digestion, respiration, etc. Setting the intentions for bedtime can enable your body to focus on healing or repairing any areas that have been broken down or harmed during the day due to toxic energy. Setting intentions is as simple as thinking or, even more powerful, speaking the plan to do this.

While your physical body is at rest, your soul is free to move on to other activities that do not need a physical presence. This is the time that most of you exercise your ability to return to the other side energetically.

Although many of you delve into other timelines that you create through dreams. This is a space in which you are able to try out different outcomes of actions you may not be courageous enough to take during your waking hours in the physical bodies of this lifetime–But I digress.

The state of sleep brings your body into a harmonious place where it can set aside the challenges of the day and focus entirely on repairing any systems that need bringing into alignment. The blockages, on the other hand, remain unless you clear them before resting. In order that you may take full advantage of any overnight healing, it is crucial that you release any energetic blockages before sleeping.

So, sleep restores you as much as possible (due to blockages) to your original perfect condition. Your soul joins together with Source to strengthen your ability to see your overall plan. Unfortunately, as your soul travels back into the veiled existence where you currently operate, it loses much of the message and only retains a deep knowing, a feeling of sorts. You can request to keep more of these messages in your waking hours–you need only to ask. Because of free will and the promise not to interfere, you must make requests to receive assistance. But with that said, constant communication is available to help guide you and keep you from falling into places of unnecessary suffering. Your daily travels should be filled with joy and adventure, not depression, struggle, and sorrow.

Learning and accepting that your world is created from a place of illusions will begin to make clear that the only reality that exists is on the "other side of the veil." Eternity is your true existence; where you think you are now is more like a dream state where you are able to work out the lessons and experiences of duality. And, of course, to come to a clear understanding of the importance of always choosing love to experience joy and peace.

But again, I digress. There is so much and yet so little that you need to know. Simply choosing love over fear will lead you to the path you are best suited, and to live your best adventure.

But during your travels you need the best operating version of your physical body. It serves as your outer protective shell for your soul while your ego mind operates this protective shell. I am comparing or describing it in this way to allow you to comprehend that this "body suit" you wear is filled with "technology" that has the ability to alert you to so many things. For example, the nervous system that indicates the temperature is too hot or too cold. Or the existence of chronic pain to alert you to potential damage to a particular area of your body. This body suit is capable of sensing danger energetically. For example, when you walk into a room, and it just doesn't feel right.

I could compare your lack of knowledge as to how your body suit works to not knowing all of the cool things an iPhone does. In other words, you can do the basics with your iPhone (or other smartphone device), but there are so many unexplained little extras that could make your life easier if you knew how they worked.

Think of this section as the part that gives you access to some of those physical body suit extras that you may or may not know of...

Epidemiology studies chronic pain. Let's look at what chronic pain can inform you of pertaining to the health of your body. For example, back pain. When you first feel discomfort is the moment your systems are alerting you to pause and reflect and release. If you have been under stressful conditions, absorbing negative emotions, suffering through life's ups and downs, then you would have accumulated quite a bit of toxic energy within your physical body. Remember, your body consists of atoms that huddle together at different frequencies to create your body suit. When other lower, denser frequencies that are slow moving coagulate within the framework of your physical body, they create barriers, blockages, and problems. When your system can no longer freely move energy throughout it, then necessary nutrients are unable to reach their planned destinations. This can literally appear as swelling or inflammation in an area that is an obvious blockage. When the body releases these blockages, the energy is able to move again and continue on its path to maintaining wellness.

This "smart body function" which we will refer to as SBF is an alert system to tell you to pause, reflect, and release. Pausing from your physical activity, reflecting on what is going on in your current moment and how it is affecting you, and setting the intention to let go and release these emotions and toxic energy to clear the path for normal functioning. An energy healer can also give you one-on-

one guidance in how to release these energies. Use discernment in choosing someone.

Another SBF includes having the ability to know when something is good for you or should be avoided. This has been called muscle testing. There are many videos online that can show you how to use this technique. To explain it here briefly: Muscle testing is the ability of your body to use magnetic energy to communicate with you by giving you a yes or no answer. It can be used to choose healthier foods and healthier products for personal care. As you develop a clear communication path with Myself, Source, it can also be used to communicate. But this is best only when you have clearly made a choice to leave behind the influence of your ego mind, and this takes much practice. Please note, I am not a fortune teller, and muscle testing should not be used as a means to make decisions on larger life choices. You should always trust your inner guidance for this.

The next SBF (smart body function) might not surprise you, but you may need to be reminded of its relevance in your current world. Discernment is something that you all struggle to master. It seems that every day someone is able to lie without being detected. Many try to use verbal cues that people give, or physical evidence that they are misleading you, but there is a much simpler way of locating the deceiver. Muscle testing can be used to know if the information you are receiving is true/yes or false/no. You can't ask about the messenger, but you can use this to discern the message. To clarify, you should not ask if the person is lying. Instead you should ask, "Is the information

I just received from this person true/yes or false/no?" This keeps you from judging the person, and instead you discern the information.

NOTE: Everything you do should be in the highest good for all, therefore judging a person/the messenger is not in the highest good. Judging the message is in the highest good.

The next SBF might amaze you, or it might not. Have you ever had a tingly feeling in your face? Your hands? Your leg? What could this possibly be trying to communicate to you? Lack of oxygen. Yes, your body is trying to tell you to breathe. Inhale in the right side of your nose while holding closed the left side. Then exhale out of the left side while holding the right side. Then reverse breathing in left, exhaling right while holding the opposite nostril. Do this 8 times slowly, and you will rebalance the oxygen levels in your body. This also works for any body part that has the "falling asleep/pins and needles" sensation. This works every time. This procedure is great for every morning routine as it helps bring into alignment your spine by diffusing oxygen up and down each side of the body by alternating the side in which you inhale and exhale. Deep breathing is cleansing for your body and is one of the quickest ways to balance chaotic, low-density emotions such as fear and anger.

The flow of clean air set with an intention of healing will instill within your physical body what is needed to create a brisk channel of energy to flush out any small blockages. Some may consider oxygen the cure to diseases such as cancer. What if? Yes, it could be that simple.

Flushing out toxic energy is the cure to everything. Just don't go overboard, keep it simple. Breathe in and out clean air filtered by plants and trees. Soak in the sun during sunrise and sunset times, and let the ocean, lakes, and streams wash away and cleanse your system. The earth provides wonderful healing modalities.

What about the SBF that involves seeing flashing lights within your eyesight? Many flock to an eye doctor, but what if it is just another alert? What could they be trying to tell you? Flashing lights signify dry eyes. Perhaps you have been in windy conditions? Or you have been focused and have not been blinking? Blinking brings moisture to the eyeball, and when you are not resting your eyes, these alerts will force you to blink and pause. To clear the lights, try blinking your eyes several times, then closing them for a minute or longer. This should end the flashing lights.

Continuing on to the next SBF, we have listed several alerts that your body gives out, but what about special dual functions? Let's start with memory. How does your ego mind determine what information should stay readily available within your memory bank and what information will be harder to retain or pull forward? You. You are the soul calling the shots, you are the one operating this smart body and giving instructions to the ego mind. You are your soul. Your soul is the essence within this body suit. Through thoughts and spoken words, you dictate what and how memories are stored. Just like your favorite numbers stored on your iPhone for easy retrieval, you have the ability to signify what information should be recalled easily and quickly.

How? It is so easy it will become one of your favorite SBFs. You just think it. For example, when you need to remember someone's phone number, you set the intention that you will need this information often and then repeat the information. That's it. Try it now. Think of a 6-8 digit number and write it down. Then tell yourself, "I will need this information often." Then read aloud the number several times. Wait a few minutes and then quiz yourself. It should work.

Another outstanding SBF is the ability to see opportunities before they appear before you. It is a dream technique that is quite simple. Before going to bed, take a few moments to make this request: "I would like to remember any visions or dreams that will be opportunities in my near future. Please show them to me in a form or vision that I can easily understand and relate." Over the next few nights as you sleep, keep a journal. When you first wake in the morning, record anything you remember. If you wake in the middle of the night, do the same. Record everything. Then each day read over your notes, and you should be able to connect the dots to see what is coming your way. This is the way your soul can leave imprints or messages within your ego mind from the other side of the veil as your soul travels back and forth. It often does this, but without your request for assistance in remembering this information, the information is buried deep within your memory because it was derived from your dream state.

Most of you like to dream, and in doing so you spend time playing out scenarios on other timelines. This method helps you work out emotions that tend to pile up within you in this timeline of events. When you spend most of your time creating more illusions to counteract the emotions created from events in this illusion, you waste valuable time that could be generating priceless guidance and information to help you evolve and live a vibrant, joyful life.

You can avoid this debacle by releasing emotions before bedtime, clearing out any toxic energy, and setting the intention to use your dream state hours to receive and remember divine guidance. Connecting with Myself, Source, will enable you to stay protected, and you will only receive benevolent messages. As you begin this process, it is strongly recommended that you stay with the most trusted energies to guide you until you have become a master of discernment. This is not to frighten you, only to encourage caution. You should never give up your freedom/free will. Benevolent energies will only guide you to think and act in your highest good and the highest good of all. They will never command you to think or do anything due to the gift of free will.

Another SBF you might enjoy learning about is the ability of the smart body to project your energy towards those around you, inducing an immediate change. Now this is where you need to know that what you do comes back to you. Some refer to this as Karma. Use your powers for benevolence.

Now, let me explain. When you send out love and light and

other powerful energies to those around you, they are received. The energies can even be put in foods and drinks. If someone cooks a meal with love and joy, the cells of the food will be balanced and will be better received by the physical host body. The body will be able to digest the food and use it to rebuild cells that need repair or replacement. But if the cooking was done in the midst of anger and fear, then the cells will be misaligned and even fragmented. When these cells enter the body, they are often rejected and cause stomach pain and problems within the excretory system. Many people bless their food before eating, and this is a good start. Something to add is a request to have any toxic, non-balanced energy to be transmuted into the frequency of love and light to enable the cells to regain their alignment before being eaten. This all might sound just incredibly insane to you, but what if? It's worth speaking a few words from the heart just in case, wouldn't you agree? You have nothing to lose except time in the closest restroom if the food contains toxic energy.

Water is also highly affected by mood, music, and chemicals. Setting an intention of healing to your glass of water before drinking can change the molecular structure of the water. Look it up, even your scientists agree with this!

But back to projecting energy. It goes both ways. Other people's energy also affects you. For example, when your close friend or family member is in a terrible mood, it often brings you into a similar state of being. They can do this just by walking into the room. So with this in mind, it is important to remember not to absorb other people's low energy. Instead try to bring them up to your vibration, and if you are unable or unwilling to do this, give them some space to protect your own energy bubble.

On to the next SBF, something that you would never have even thought was useful, but it can create big changes in your life. The time you spend trying to understand what is wrong with someone, what you think you did to create this obstacle, is often nothing to do with you. Instead they are projecting themselves on you. In other words, they see their weakness in you instead of themselves. So how does the smart body help with this?

Have you ever been in a car with someone and felt they were avoiding talking about a particular subject? Perhaps you just had a disagreement, but they are talking about everything except what happened? And you know you are not to blame—you can see that they are blaming you for something that you did not do, but you feel stuck. You are avoiding the conversation because you do not want to make things worse, and you know that they would not get your side of it. The point would be lost. What do you do?

You rely on your SBF guidance. You think in your head, *please Source, give me the words to say in this situation. Let me leave this person better than I found them.* Then stay silent and wait for the thoughts to arrive. These thoughts will guide you slowly and confidently as to what to say and when to be quiet and let them respond. The difficult part might be following the guidance exactly. For if you go off script, you will be on your own.

It might be helpful to practice this a few times in situations that are more easily improved by following the guidance. Maybe ask for this assistance the next time you are planning to enter a store or a group of people that you find challenging to be around. Ask and you shall receive.

And yes, this SBF is more of a combination feature. It relies on your physical body to alert you to the uncomfortable feeling and the Soul's direct contact with Spirit to convey the messages of assistance needed.

And this begins to show you the importance of how everything links together (Body, Mind, Soul, and Spirit), creating the perfect situation for you – that is, if you know the features available.

There are more, but perhaps I will save those for another time.

To continue, we should look at other ways to maintain the appropriate highest functioning condition of your physical body and software/mind.

It certainly helps to maintain a size and weight that enables quick movement and the least amount of disabling alerts. These alerts include digestion problems, acne, dizziness, and more. To avoid these symptoms, destabilizing foods and drinks must be avoided.

This is where programming becomes essential. Let's take two examples that you can imagine.

The first involves a person that has been programmed by television, colorful food labels, and friends telling them over and over again that sugar is a treat and is something to be enjoyed and brought out on special occasions. Our second example is programmed by experiencing life away from media influence. Perhaps they live on an island where they grow their own fresh vegetables and fruits. This person has been programmed by their lifestyle to appreciate the abundance of colorful fruits and vegetables, and they celebrate by consuming special foods prepared for generations with love by family members.

The difference is obvious. Being programmed to joyfully eat healthy without being exposed to sugar and other toxic chemicals makes living easy. Of course, most of you do not live on a secluded island. Instead you have spent your life surrounded by the first example's programming.
The good news is that your system can be reset. And this is what you may find to be the key to losing weight and maintaining a size that operates and functions best.

Your taste buds will need to be reset to enjoy new tastes and to reject sugary sweetness. This can be achieved by following a new routine involving the foods you consume for one week. Yes, it only takes one week to reprogram your taste buds. Exposing yourself to only healthy fresh fruits and vegetables and replacing sugary drinks with water will enable your system to pivot away from past foods that you craved.

In fact, after a few weeks, the sugary foods will no longer taste good to you.

But this is truly the easy part. The difficulty remains in the daily bombardment of sugary ads on television, your social media, and the programming that still remains within your friends and family. What if I were to tell you that simply challenging yourself to set the pace for everyone else can help you stay ahead of all of those temptations? It is a mindset, a programming of the mind that will need to hear daily reminders to stay on target.

By now you are understanding the power of thought and the triple power of the spoken word to your always listening cells. You can easily convince your physical body/ego mind that celery is a treat just by speaking it aloud. Whenever you start to slip, remember the process of reprogramming. Remind yourself that sugar is not a treat. Sugar is harmful. Sugar is a poison to your body. Why would you eat poison?

Removing sugary snacks and drinks from your home is also recommended. And as you remind yourself that these foods are toxic to your system, it will become much easier to replace them with healthy options.

It's somewhat odd that so many have become comfortable feeding themselves and their children these toxic chemicals. Making this change should not overwhelm anyone. This is one simple change that would relieve you all of so much suffering. And after making these changes, you will quickly crave the sweetness of a delicious apple or some other piece of fruit.

Pharmacology - Drugs - Prescriptions - Treatments

These are words to pause and reflect on–asking how your life is intertwined with these ways of dealing with sickness, painful symptoms, and disease. Treating an illness does not cure an illness. There are many prescriptions written by well-intentioned doctors that do not understand how the physical body actually functions. Most do not understand because they have not been shown how energies coagulate to create blockages. And they certainly have zero interest in removing these energies that they are unaware of.

You have the opportunity to try these methods for yourself. Nothing ventured, nothing gained. And what do you have to lose? Illness, suffering, high cost of prescriptions that have many side effects.

Again, as a reminder. Energy can not be destroyed. It can be transmuted or moved. You are made entirely of energy, atoms clustered together in the form of your physical body. The cancers, the cysts, the debris that clogs your systems consist of lower, denser, slow vibrating energies. These are the energies that create blockages that keep everything from freely moving to maintain each complementary system within your smart body.

The key is to keep everything moving and to remove blockages as soon as they appear before they have time to grow and cause more damage.

As time goes on, your body ages, or so you think it must age and continue breaking down. But this is not true.

It is true that your body must physically grow to adulthood, but the rapid progression after age 30 is not necessary. To alleviate the symptoms of aging, you need only to realize that it is an illusion that your ego mind has been scripted to move in that direction.

What if? What if, for example, you no longer thought those thoughts. What if you realized that you are in control, and your cells are directed by what you think and speak. Your body replaces itself through regeneration of cells constantly. Over and over again it regenerates, but through your programming you have directed it to begin the aging process. And where did you learn of this aging process? By watching those before you age, yes, of course. But also by the marketing that sells products, the surgeons that remove wrinkles, etc.

So, what do you do? You simply let go of the previous ways of thinking and directing your cells. You begin to communicate the truth. And what is the truth? The truth is that you can direct your cells to revert back to the original blueprint of your body. The original plans are stored within your DNA awaiting your instructions.

At this point let's stop to consider that you along with everyone else gave up. You surrendered your sovereignty. Perhaps you think it is easier for someone else to make decisions for you? Or you felt incompetent? Or maybe you thought it was too great a responsibility?

But look around you, is there truly anyone that is better than yourself to decide what is best for you?

When you leave these decisions to others, they do not put you first. And greed steps in and makes adjustments that openly benefit only one small group of people. And over time this group becomes smaller and smaller.

Each of you is capable, each is divine, each houses a spark within them that knows what is best for everyone, including themselves.

Free will is a gift that each of you were born with and few of you actively use to your benefit. Free will allows you to make choices all day every day. And yet, over and over again, you choose poorly. You choose unhealthy diets, you choose unhealthy partners, you choose deceit and greed over truth and abundance for all.

Your smart body has many functions, but like any computer system, it is only as smart or helpful as the programmer. And in this case, you are the programmer. You call the shots. You utilize your free will moment to moment to make decisions, including the ones that affect how your smart body functions and how well it is maintained.

Studies show that your health and well-being are affected greatly by the amount of exercise you participate in on a daily basis. It often says that your cardio/heart health is contingent upon you getting enough strenuous movement to raise your heart rate. In your society it is argued that a busy, quick-paced lifestyle is healthiest. And this seems to have been taken too far. Many of your days are spent hurrying from one event or activity to the next, competing with your peers to produce a greater amount of work completed instead of taking the time to pause and reflect and study to create the best outcomes. Instead your outcomes are driven by money, whereas a better way would be to focus your intention and energy on producing quality long-lasting outcomes that benefit the greater good. Yes, for the most part you have all lost your way, and this contributes to the breakdown of your smart body in the form of stress.

Stress-induced activities, conversations, movies, music, and even your thoughts parade about you causing a longer-lasting detrimental effect than you could possibly imagine. And what is the cause? Fear.

Yes, fear. Fear of failure. Fear of loss. Fear of not being loved. You have been programmed to operate in a state of fear. A continuous stream of fearful thoughts or feelings/emotions keep you in a fight or flight mode creating stress. It is a wonder that you still live past the age of childhood, especially since these fears are pressed upon your children beginning earlier and earlier. Think about the unnecessary fears that your children are burdened with constantly. The fear of pleasing you instead of loving to be accepted as perfect souls by you. So many fears revolving around safety and security, sports competitions, school accomplishments, fitting in with friends, and the list goes on and on.

Children are perfect. And when they are nurtured and accepted and loved, they thrive without needing discipline. Guidance is needed but not punishment.

Children need your protection and love, not your judgment and disapproval.

But let's get back to your smart body and the questions you may have concerning how much movement, or what you call exercise, is necessary. Movement does more than just keep your heart healthy. It stretches and utilizes muscles, while also helping maintain your ability to move and partake in fun activities. It is also a great mode of transportation, walking or running. Although walking is best. The expression, "use it or lose it" does apply here. If you are out of practice, then you will find it difficult to move. Stretching and moving your body in different directions helps you stay flexible and keeps your smart body in better physical shape and in a state of readiness for any adventures that may come your way. It only makes sense to keep yourself flexible and strong just in case a great opportunity presents itself to do something that requires more than sitting and watching television.

So, the amount needed equates to the type of adventure you would like to be able to participate in. Your time here is brief, I would recommend being ready for anything! After all, you came all this way for a grand adventure! Don't let your lack of readiness hinder your enjoyment of your experience.

As time continues along, this adventure seems to move more quickly every day. Slowing down and taking time to truly take in the experience that you have come to have will lead you closer and closer to your original plan.

Everything around you serves as a distraction. You arrived alone with your guides/angels to assist you on a journey that is yours alone. You did not make reservations on Earth to meet up with your friends and attend a great party. You made a plan, we made a plan together for you to evolve, to grow in your consciousness and understanding of duality and the benefits of always creating from a place of love. Those that cross your path may benefit from your interactions, and you may benefit from their participation in your experience, but in the end your experience is solely yours. You are granted free will to pick and choose along the way, enabling you to make decisions that either choose a more difficult path or a divine path. It is always up to you. No one else should ever make these decisions for you, and when you are tempted to grant someone else the opportunity to choose for you, you will have failed to realize your ability and your sovereignty.

And as you are granted this type of existence, you must come to respect that all other souls traveling along this journey are also recipients of the same free will and should be left space to make their own choices.

Of course, children do require more protection and guidance, but only in regards to survival in the physical world. They also should be granted free thoughts and to allow their imaginations to create from a place of good intentions. Mistakes will be made, but that is all they are – mistakes. Learning to pivot and make better choices is always the reaction desired. This is truly simple. Choose love over fear – always.

Your smart body creates a vehicle of sorts for you to meander around your environment and create experiences for yourself. It enables you to interact with other souls and sometimes produces situations that call for you to strive to remain without judgment. Yes, often you will see qualities in others that you do not like, but you are not responsible for their qualities or their actions. No need to remind you, but here it is – you have more than enough to focus on pertaining to your own qualities/actions and behaviors without even thinking about anyone else's. Put your energy into grooming yourself to be the best, most compassionate recipient of experiences. Without judging, learn to respect the behaviors of others and focus entirely on your behavior, response, or reaction instead.

Think as if each person in your life is writing their own life story, and you are a character in their book. My advice is to be the best character possible. You have your own book to write – focus on this instead.

And how does this relate to your smart body? It benefits your health and well-being when you have discovered the best way to just be. By leaving all of your body's daily functions up to your ego mind and using the guidance from your higher self to lessen the toxic energy that comes in contact with your smart body, you will maintain your body, you will lengthen its age, and you will enjoy its health and wellness greatly in your daily travels. Not to mention the great role model you will become for others to avoid suffering and finally enjoy life.

And now perhaps you would like to learn one more helpful smart body function. Like the iPhone, the more you practice these, the more helpful they become.

Let's begin with your ability to cross information from one life to another. This is not your first time here, and you have collected many experiences to build upon in this lifetime. Your DNA stores all of this information, although some of it can become unhelpful. For example, if you drowned in a previous life, you may have carried that fear of water into this experience. Look at the fears you have and work to let go of those traumas. Realize that fears are illusions, just as death is an illusion, for your soul is eternal. The only thing that stops or ends is the use of this body suit/smart body. This you leave behind to meld back into the earth's energy as you return to a higher dimension.

The positive to carrying this information is it creates talents and abilities that you may have worked lifetimes to establish such as painting, singing, writing, etc. Look at what you consider your natural talents and see if any of those are activities that you would like to continue in this lifetime. Oftentimes they are part of a greater plan, and this is the lifetime for you to use those talents to create from the heart to make great steps in your spiritual growth. Sharing these talents with others should grant you a deep peace, giving you the sign that you need to know if you are on the correct path. And what is the correct path? The path to your journey home. That is the path that everyone eventually finds themselves following, and the earlier you discover your footing, the earlier you will be able to enjoy your journey.

There is no need to rush and no need to run. Time only exists temporarily. You have forever to reach home, and there is much to see along the way.

How do you know for sure that you are on the right path? Does your smart body tell you? In some ways, yes, and others not exactly. The nervous system assists you to remain out of the way of danger for the most part, but your ego mind does not have your divine plan or access to it.

The only way to gain access to this guidance is through your soul via spirit. Spirit is the liaison between yourself and Me, Source. Spirit fills the role of the translator of sorts by giving you words you can understand that relate to your daily experiences that I, Source, do not find applicable. To better understand this, remember that as Source, I am the frequency of love and therefore do not know fear, anger, hate, etc. You are currently in a dualistic environment, and Spirit is needed to convey messages that you can understand from a source that does not experience what you experience. The awareness is there, but without the emotion. Without the experience of existing within a physical body constantly battling an ego mind, I, Source, can only imagine from a place of love what this experience is like. Admiration is great for the ability to delve into such a low density environment and still create from a place of love while being so bombarded with hatred and negativity.

And how does your smart body function help you with all of this? Your physical body captures all of the details of your current surroundings, creating a database for your soul to tap into.

This database is used to compare and contrast information from your previous lifetimes/experiences. It helps create channels of information within your mind/software that can be utilized to help you in certain situations that were planned before you arrived.

For example, you may find that some activities seem easier for you than others. This is because previously stored information creates channels that your ego mind can easily gain access to during this life experience. It will seem more natural because it will not be surrounded by all of the unnecessary details that were collected along with the learning that was captured for the activity.

In other words, you may have a remembering of playing the piano but not remember the people involved and possible traumatic events that surrounded your previous life experience. Letting go of the traumas and just keeping the learned abilities is in your highest good moving forward.

And how do you do this? You merely ask. From a place of genuine heartfelt curiosity, you can request to bring forth the knowing and understanding of these abilities so that you may use them in this current experience.

There is so much for you to learn about this smart body of yours. But for now, this is the overall picture to get you started. As more of you begin to understand what the bundle of atoms known as a physical body is and does, I will share more.

For now, this is it. This is the starting point for you to begin letting go of previous programming and open up to the possibilities of finally understanding and receiving the truth. You are love, you are loved. Life is for experiencing and creating from a place of love while experiencing the duality that exists in this place you call Earth. I hope you will rise to meet Me, to seek the guidance that is available for you to thrive. I am here. I am waiting, and I have much to share.

Much love and admiration,
Source

Takeaway quotes from this letter from Source...

"Your ego mind is in charge of the daily activities."

"So, there is a purpose for the ego mind. It also helps protect what we will refer to the physical body as the SB (smart body).
You could say the SB is the outer shell of a computer or robot. And the ego mind is the software that runs it."

"...your ego mind does not have the ability to guide you in terms of morality or benevolence. It does not understand the difference between what is right and what is wrong."

"The ego mind does not love. It only grabs information and stores it and brings it to the surface to remind you of the past."

"And here is the interesting thing. The ego mind is the producer of information to help you analyze situations. It creates a mental environment for you to compare and contrast information to help you decide what to do – but it is based entirely upon bits of information gathered, unrelated at the time to this decision and without the big picture being available to be seen."

"What if you were to rely on another Source and accept the guidance from this Source that is always choosing for the highest good?"

"...once one energetic atom becomes lodged, others will attach causing a type of coagulation that creates a blockage. These blockages impede the flow of energy, including everything your body needs to stay well (nutrients for cell repair, water for energy flow, etc.)."

"Ridding the physical body of these negative energies frees up the space and pathways for your energy to regulate and maintain your bodily functions. Your body uses oxygen and water to flush toxins from your systems."

"So, what should you do to remove it? It is as simple as setting the intention and energetically waving away these clumps of coagulated low vibrational energy. Since they are moving at such a slow vibrational pace, when you increase your overall vibration (raise your frequency), your overall energy will shake the stagnant energy loose, and it should be set free."

"The effects of sound on your system are enormous."

"Every sound that you come in contact with tries to penetrate your protective outer energetic boundary. Many refer to this as your aura, an energy field that surrounds your body..."

"When you are physically still in a hypnotic state, your soul becomes not the observer but the influencer. It then gains full control and can relay information from your energetic being that is fully aware to your mind that is installed in your physical body. It can be a pathway to communicate with your soul."

"Why is this important? This is where your true divine guidance is derived. It needs a pathway that is not interrupted by your ego mind."

"And there is no reason for forgiveness, there is no sin, just error. Error easily corrected."

"And what does this have to do with healing? It is the foundation for healing. First you must accept and create space for dismissal of errors. You must allow yourself to accept that you are good. You are love, and you are light. As long as you hold onto the thoughts that box you in as imperfect, you will never see yourself as whole and healed. By seeing yourself as anything less than how you were originally created is to give space to the illusion that you could actually be less than, or in your terms, ill."

"Healing yourself is the beginning to healing the world."

"What more could you ask for?" (From following the guidance from Source.)

"Perhaps stability? Peace in your life? Everlasting joy? Oh, but these are the gifts that are yours at the very moment that you extend them to others."

"So together, energy, frequency, and vibration determine your overall health and well-being..."

"Within your DNA, all of the appropriate instructions, guidelines, blueprints, etc. are stored, and your ego mind has access to this information. Your ego mind as the software of your body just needs your green light "go" request to enable the communication to begin. This is why I have referred to your body as the "smart body." It already knows what to do with such frequency requests, but until now you have not known that you needed to do this."

"...your thoughts are much more powerful than you know, and your spoken words have the ability to wreak havoc on not only yourself but others."

"You have the inner guidance/coach always with you striving for your best outcome. Perhaps it's time that you gave it a chance."

"Choose substance over frivolity. Choose happiness over trying to impress someone else. Be authentic, be present, just be. A smart body has the ability to run itself, but the soul will need direction. For your soul's eternal stake in the everlasting, choose substance. Always choose substance."

Other books available:

Love
Advice
Raising Children
Smart Body
Now
Healing
Guidance
Co-parenting
Free Will
Salvation
Conversations
Invisible to Visible
Duality
Solutions
Smart Body II
Faith vs Religion

Please help me share these
messages to inspire others to live
a more joyful life by sharing this
book with a friend.

For other books written with
messages from Source and for
daily/weekly messages, please visit
my website for social media links
or email me directly.

Thank you!

Love to you on your journey.

Carrington Allen
CarringtonAllen.com
carringtonsemail@gmail.com

Please use the following pages to
begin to journal any guidance you
receive from Source. A few quiet
moments to pause and listen and
record what you hear through your
thoughts can start you on your path
to an amazing tomorrow. Often
I would begin by writing down
a question and then wait for the
answer. Whatever comes to mind,
write it down...this is where the
adventure begins.

Notes:

Notes:

Notes:

Notes:

Notes:

Notes: